Essentials Oils for Weight Loss

A Few Drops a Day Will Keep the Fat Bulges Away

I0427756

Disclaimer

Summary

You probably started this New Year with a resolution to lose weight and that may seem impossible to achieve. The fact is, excess fat itself is not a disease, but it may become the root cause of many problems, including health risks, lack of confidence and social isolation. It is a widespread problem, and researchers believe that nearly one-third of adults (approximately 35% of total population) living in the United States are obese. These 78 million people and many others around the world, everyday try various weight loss measures including exercise, diet, and medicines. Some individuals go to the extent of surgical procedures to get rid of this traumatic problem.

These procedures may pose serious threats to your overall wellbeing. However, if you are looking for a permanent and safe solution to cellulite, this book has everything you need to know. Weight loss can be utterly easy with essential oil therapies and treatments.

'Essential Oils for Weight Loss' will introduce you to a take-action/practical approach to the perfect body shape. What you will find and learn in this book:

1. Know and measure the extra weight that you may be carrying
2. Understanding the health risks of excess weight
3. A comparison between natural remedies and surgical procedures
4. The reason why essential oils have a positive impact on physical health
5. A detailed description of each natural oil, its uses, benefits and extraction methods
6. Usage of oils to enhance skin's natural glow
7. Miraculous beauty tips
8. Losing weight to overcome health related problems such as diabetes, poor digestion, and cardiac diseases.
9. Easy essential oil body wraps to lose inches in weeks

In short, this book has all the information about pure essential oils and their powerful non-invasive properties to reduce weight. Continue reading to unveil secrets that have never been disclosed before.

Contents

Introduction: Getting Rid of Bad Fat

Obesity is a rapidly growing problem that is now a concern of many international non-government organizations including World Health Organization (WTO). The recent government statistics have revealed shocking obesity trends; nearly one in three U.S.citizens are overweight or obese. It is no more a problem that is confined to a particular gender or age. The studies have shown almost an equal ratio of obesity issues in both men and women. The reason why local and international health communities are alarmed is the health risks imposed by this epidemic.

To overcome the problem, scientists have been introducing new ways of weight loss such as medicines and advanced surgical procedures. On the other hand, everyday new kinds of exercise machines are advertised, giving new hopes to the struggling individuals who are battling against this ugly truth. However, the results are either not long lasting, or come with a variety of side effects that are even more harmful than fat itself.

Due to the evident disadvantages of mainstream conventional methods, doctors and other health professionals are shifting towards alternative medicine and aromatherapies. Essential oils have been scientifically proven to offer natural solutions to treat core health and wellness issues. While healthy eating and regular exercising should always be a part of a healthy lifestyle, naturally extracted oils will boost the metabolism, which is one great way to shed extra pounds.

Know your Weight: Check your BMI

A healthy body has nothing to do with the impossible-to-achieve Barbie doll figure; it is about maintaining a weight that is proportional to your height, age, and gender. So exactly what is the perfect amount of body fat you should aim for? How do you find out whether you are overweight or not? It may sound tricky, but by measuring your BMI (Body Mass Index), you will know exactly where you stand and how far you have to go ahead with your weight loss journey. BMI is a standard gauge to whether a person is overweight, underweight, or possesses a perfect proportion of fat.

The first step to calculate BMI is to convert pounds into kilograms and measure height in terms of meters. To change pounds into kilograms, divide your total weight by 2.2.Then check your height in meters, by dividing the total inches by 39.37. Now multiply the result by itself. Then divide your weight in kilograms by the figure that you have just calculated. Here is a solved numerical example to assist your calculations.

If you are 65 inches tall, weighing about 180 pounds, your BMI figures should look like this:

180lbs / 2.2 = 81.81 kg

65 inches/ 39.37 = 1.65 meter

1.65 X 1.65= 2.7225

81.81 kg / 2.7225 = 30.04

Reference range:

Less than 19: Underweight

19 to 25: Normal

25 to 30: Overweight

More than 30: Obese

Consider yourself lucky if your BMI falls between the normal range, if you do not, take things seriously for there is nothing more precious than good health.

Measuring the Risk of Excess Fat

Carrying extra or unwanted body fat does not only look undesirable, but it also makes a person feel bad. Such people usually feel the lack of energy in performing the daily household chores. Since the work becomes an ordeal, they even tend to lose their temper and get frustrated easily. While all these symptoms are behavioral, their physical health is also endangered. Excess weight is one of the most commonly known reasons of some serious conditions, including cardiac arrest.

Childhood obesity often results in long-term health problems, as those who are obese as children are likely to develop health related issues at an early age. Experts suggest that being overweight can increase your risk for high blood pressure, diabetes, high cholesterol, stroke, heart disease, and cancer. In the later chapters of this book, you will find ways and dietary tips that can help in easing the health hazards.

Natural Remedies vs. Surgical Procedures

When it comes to effectiveness of various weight loss methods, people tend to compare every aspect of the procedure. The generally concerned areas are cost, efficiency, side effects, and application.

Surgical Procedures

Considering the costs of operations like tummy tucks and gastric sleeves, it is not advised that you make changes to your digestive system. Although it offers instant results (mostly within three months), its after-effects can be very critical. The risks involved in a bypass surgery include: allergic reactions to chemically-produced medicines, blood clotting, pregnancy complications and stroke during the process.

Natural Remedies

On the contrary, you have the option of natural herbs and oils that can influence your hunger and appetite without causing any damage to your body. It regulates your emotions, senses and feelings, which is one of the causes of obesity. You will be surprised to know that essential oils are available for less than half the price of many weight reduction tablets sold in pharmacies. Read on to know more details of essential oils and their various health benefits.

Causes of Weight Gain

Lack of Water

On an average, for each pound of weight, the human body requires approximately 0.5 ounces of water. This minimum threshold is necessary for the body to function properly and flush out all toxins that are entered in our body through environment, food, smoking and consumption of chemically produced beverages. There are many people who do not like the taste of simple water, and therefore do not intake more than 4 to 5 glasses a day. Fortunately, there are some essential oils such as citrus fresh, which can improve the taste of water, helping you consume at least 8 glasses a day.

Poor Diet

Eating food items that lack vital nutrients creates low alkalinity, which forces the body to crave sugar. Besides that, junk food is another significant reason why obesity is becoming more common among the youth. The sugar cravings can be effectively stopped by the help of essential oils.

Lack of Nutrition

Taking supplements to compensate for the natural need of nutrients may prove to be a bad idea; after all, human-made chemical formulas cannot match the goodness of natural herbs. Herbal weight loss contains vitamins and enzymes that provide the body with adequate amounts of natural energy required.

Toxicity

Negative thought, stress, unhealthy diet and environmental pollution are a few of the reasons why there may be toxins in our body. These toxic remains are stored in our body in a form of fat that does not burn easily. While drinking fresh juices and water can drain toxicity, oils that are rich in citrus considerably eliminate waste from the body. This thorough detoxification process also helps in quitting smoking and overcoming addictions.

Lack of Exercise

Due to a slow metabolism in bodies that are loaded with unwanted fat, you may feel lethargic when it comes to physical activities. This sluggish behavior can also be treated with oils that give you a sense of instant energy by uplifting your spirits. Certain oils can also be used to fix emotional instabilities that hinder calorie-burning processes.

Lack of Sleep

This might come to you as a surprise, but yes, sleep disorders might also be one of the reasons why you have extra bulges around your waist. Sleeping less means you will feel a lack of energy that is crucial for a balanced endocrine (hormonal) system. It does not only disturb the digestion's organism, but also makes you eat more to reimburse the energy needed for an active life. Thanks to the magic of aromatherapy, insomnia will turn into a good night's sleep.

Hormonal Imbalance

Hormones are chemical receptors that control the communication system of our body. A misbalance of hormones in the endocrine system results in unwanted or rapid weight gain. This influences cravings, metabolism, and fat distribution. When these glands are secreted into the bloodstream, it works with the immune and nervous system to regulate and generate various emotions.

People who are obese can find it difficult to work out, exercise, or indulge in a demanding physical activity. This behavior further slows down their fat burning process, causing body to restore more amounts of fat every day.

Use of certain oils can help in calming stressed nerves, resulting in a more balanced or normalized eating habits.

Emotional Anxiety and Depression

If you want to stay in a perfect body shape, let go of your unnecessary worries. Every time you are emotionally upset and feel anxiety, the Cortisol levels in your body increase, which is directly connected with the amount of fat piling up on your legs, arms and belly. It also acts adversely on nutrients that your body has accumulated over a period. Now you do not have to go for shopping or a movie to delight your senses, you can instead do that at home just by smelling the aroma of a natural herb.

Emotional Eating

Emotional eating refers to the cravings or temptations to eat more during a certain emotional state. Many people tend to eat more to counter or repress negative thoughts and emotions. Eating stimulates happy cells in our body, which in turn stabilizes mood and keeps depression and stress at bay. Occasionally, when a bad day or trauma strikes, people tend to nibble more than ordinary days.

This eating disorder is a major cause of obesity. Experts suggest that in more than 75% of cases, the cause of overeating is emotional eating disorder. This abnormality is stemmed from anger, loneliness, frustration, stress, depression, anxiety, and a low self-esteem. Similarly, people who lack confidence in general also tend to eat more than people who are confident about their visual appearance.

Thyroid Imbalance

Not many people are aware of the fact that thyroid-secreted hormones normalize immune function, body temperature, emotions, and the digestive system, which has drastic impacts on an individual's ability to reduce or gain weight. Essential oils can also repair damage to this small gland at the base of your neck. Other medical conditions like hypothyroidism and ovary syndromes can also be eased (if not cured) by applying and inhaling herbal oils.

Prescribed Medications

If you are using any prescribed pharmaceutical drugs like birth control pills, antibiotics, tranquilizers, antidepressants and lithium, there are chances of you gaining weight rapidly. Chemicals in these medicines produce toxins and probiotic deficiency that radically contribute towards abnormal weight gain. Unlike artificial medical substances, oils extracted from herbs do not affect adversely on your body.

Aging

As we age, our ability to produce hormones, absorb nutrients, generate enzymes and maintain metabolic rates depletes. This natural aging process results in weight gain along with other physiological changes. Due to lack of energy, a person may not be able to exercise and physically exert. Aging of course cannot be reversed, but natural herbs and oils can slow down the process of aging and improve the quality of life.

Essential Oils: An Effective Weight Loss Solution

If your New Year resolution is to get back in shape and look your best, and all other weight loss plans that you have tried are stalled, you need to explore some fine ingredients and herbal extracts that will burn fat as you apply and smell it. Not only this, it also reduces the stress caused by today's hustle and bustle of life. Even with all the willpower in the world, there comes a time when cravings get out of hand and soon you find yourself in a pastry shop. However, these oils and scents will kill all urges and curb those chocolate fantasies.

Inhaling scents can reduce the appetite to help you stay away from unwanted calories. Essential oils work directly on the hypothalamus gland, which regulates appetite by sending hunger signals to the brain. When it is activated, you hardly feel the craving for extra nibbling.

Caution: Safety Precautions

Oils and scents should always be used carefully as they may trigger or stimulate an additional desire to eat. The trick is to smell the aroma enough so that you are no longer tempted to eat. It is advised that you keep switching from one flavor to another because naturally, we do not crave for the same thing repeatedly. Just as we like variety on the dining table, there must be a variety of scents used for effective results. It is always helpful to understand the safety precautions before using or applying essential oils.

Abortifacient Substances

Abortifacient refers to the substances, chemicals, and herbs that have the tendency to induce an abortion. Although there is not enough clinical data available on the subject, however, some oils are known to have such characteristics including: Parsley seed, Mugwort, Rue, Pennyroyal, Thuja, Wormwood, Sassafras and Sage.

The oils listed above should never be used by pregnant women. Due to their toxic nature, it may cause an aborted fetus. However, it may be used by woman who experience prolonged menstrual cycles as the strong Emmenagogue can encourage menstruation.

Under no circumstances can this essential oil be taken orally, unless it is prescribed by a certified and licensed medical practitioner.

Aromatherapy for Elderly People

Aromatherapy is known to improve the general health of elderly people; however, one has to be careful when blending and mixing essential oils that are to be used in the therapy. Since aging often causes weakness, experts suggest a lower dilution rate for older people. In addition to that, their ongoing medication, health conditions and illnesses should also be kept in mind as it will influence the decision the essentially oil that must be used.

Nevertheless, Aromatherapy can be extremely beneficial for incapacitated patients and elderly people who are wheelchair-bound or bedridden. A gentle massage of carefully selected oils can improve blood circulation to help alleviate discomfort of staying in the same position for long hours.

Remember that essential oil therapy does not mean a patient will not need other medical treatments. It is a natural supplement to aid the healing process.

Cardiac Problems and Essential Oils

When it comes to people who are overweight or obese, the likelihood of having a heart disease automatically increases. They need to use oils that can stimulate weight loss along with the immunity to avoid heart problems. While essential oils and are known to promote good health, it may be harmful to people who already suffering from diseases, especially cardiac issues. Even if a person does not have such health problems, remember that obesity is one of the many root causes of this dangerous disease.

A heart patient should never use peppermint essential oil for its massage may trigger an increased heart pulse.

Care for Sensitive Skin

Whether it's about choosing essential oils or the daily moisturizer, people with sensitive skin are usually picky as it is a skin type that is highly prone to allergies, rash, irritations and reactions. For such people, experts suggest doing a 'patch test' before applying a new oil or oil blend.

Oils that can cause phototoxicity should be used with great care. Phototoxicity is a condition under which skin becomes extremely sensitive under the sun, especially if you work in outdoors or commute much under the sun.

With sensitive skin, one has to be extra cautious when using oils such as Orange, Wintergreen, Citronella, Peppermint, Lemongrass, Cumin, Oregano, Red and wild thyme, Lemon verbena, Basil, Parsley seed, Fennel, Ginger, Pine, Lemon, Clove, Black pepper, Cinnamon, Benzoin and Oak moss.

If you feel any irritation, sensitivity, rash or redness while using essential oils, immediately stop its usage and contact a medical professional.

Emmenagogue Herbs and Women's Health

Emmenagogues refer to the herbs and their by-products that stimulate blood flow in the uterus or pelvic area. They were traditionally used to induce menstruation in situations other than pregnancy. Some of the essential oils that promote the monthly discharge include Clary sage, Rose, Jasmine, Cinnamon, Peppermint, Ginger, Angelica, Rosemary and Sweet fennel.

Since a disturbed menstruation or menses is a major cause of abnormal or rapid weight gain, many therapists suggest the use of these oils. However, if you are pregnant or planning a child, stop its usage right away.

Nevertheless, it is helpful in treating medical conditions such as Dysmenorrhoea (a painful menstruation), Amenorrhoea (absence of menstruation), and Leucorrhoea (mucus discharge). All of these problems are extremely common in people whose BMI is more than 30.

Using Essential Oils with Children

Although essential oils have significant health benefits, it is important to remember that these are strong botanical extracts are high-concentrated and should be used carefully, especially with children. Keep the oil containers away from children's reach as these powerful compounds may prove be dangerous in case of excess or wrong usage. They should not be consumed orally unless prescribed by a doctor or healthcare expert.

Before applying on the skin, dilute it to the minimal level (1%) as children's skin is naturally sensitive and delicate. Do not leave the child unattended when inhaling the oil through steam inhalator.

Epilepsy and Use of Essential Oils

Epilepsy is a condition, which signifies a sudden malfunction of brain activity, which may cause someone to collapse and experience a loss of consciousness. It may happen due to a decrease in blood flow to the brain and mostly lasts for about 30 seconds to 2 minutes. There are different kinds of epilepsy and in some cases, the cause of a seizure is unidentified. Most people think of a seizure as a condition in which the person experiences extreme body shakes, which are rapid and uncontrollable. Not all seizures occur like that and some have mild symptoms.

Some seizures are also the result of another medical problem such as fever, low blood sugar, infection, head injury, or medicines. They can also be due to a brain problem such as a tumor.

Precaution:

Anyone who suffers or has suffered from epilepsy should avoid the following essential oils, mainly as a precaution:

Eucalyptus, Fennel, Pennroyal, Thuja, Turpentine, Rosemary, Sage, and Wormwood.

The oil, which is recommended to be used in this condition, is Frankincense. It is the oil of choice for any kind of brain disorder. It has a molecular makeup which allows it to cross the barrier between the blood and brain as it includes sesquiterpenes. This promotes brain functions such as memory and emotions. This oil has therapeutic properties such as it is antiseptic, carminative, sedative, expectorant and also slows and deepens the breath.

To apply Frankincense and prevent seizures, use a drop beneath your big toe or apply a drop of it at the base of neck and temples every night. You can also place a drop under your tongue each night.

Hepatoxicity and Essential Oils

Hepatoxicity is a condition which refers to liver toxicity. The liver is involved in carrying out many main functions for the normal functioning of the body. Most people think that the liver only detoxifies the blood but it also helps with secretion of bile, synthesis of protein and aids in carbohydrate and lipid metabolism. In this regard, some essential oils must be used with caution as they cause hepatoxicity (liver toxicity). No one should take the following essential oils orally- do not swallow- unless advised by an experienced medical practitioner. These oils cause no harm through skin absorption- such as when massaged:

Aniseed, bay, basil, buchu, cassia, cinnamon, fennel, clove, tarragon

The following oils should be avoided as they may cause liver toxicity wsen taken internally as well as in a massage blend:

Boldo Leaf, Calamus, Almond, Camphor, Horseradish, Mugwort, Jaborandi Leaf, Mustard, Rue, Sassafras, Savin, Pennyroyal, Southernwood, Nightshade, Tansy, Wintergreen, Wormwood, Wormseed, Thuja, and Stinging Nettles.

IFRA Banned Oils

Some essential oils are banned or either restricted by the International Fragrance Association because of their toxicity, certain properties and sensitizing effects. The oils that are banned are:

Calamus oil, Costus Root, Cade Oil Crude, Mustard Oil, Elecampane Oil, Fig Leaf Absolute, Peru Balsam, Savin Oil, Sassafras Oil, Stryax Gum, Tea Absolute, Verbena Oil, Wormseed, and Wormwood Oil.

Some more oils that must be used with care are not banned by the IFRA but are restricted for use due to the amount of the active ingredient contained in them, which may have possible side effects like photo toxicity, and sensitizing. These are:

Angelica Root Oil, Bergamot Oil, Cassia Oil, Bitter Orange Oil, Cinnamon Bark, Lemon Oil, Grapefruit Oil, Cumin Oil, Lime Oil, Tagetes Oil, Oak Mass Absolute, Pinaceae Oils, Rue Oil, Verbena Absolute, and Tree Mass Absolute.

Natural Toxicity of Essential Oils

You must keep in mind that while essential oils are a great source to maintain your health and benefit you with their natural properties, these are potent compounds which should always be used with extreme care. Always consult an expert aroma therapist and your medical practitioner to discuss the application of these oils, as some should not be ingested and others are advised not to be used in massage form on the body. Refrain from taking any essential oil internally especially without consulting a qualified and licensed medical practitioner. Some oils, which are toxic and should be avoided at all costs are:

Almond, Boldo, Calamus, Camphor, Cassia, Horseradish, Mugwort, Mustard, Pennyroyal, Rue, Sassafras, Savin, Thuja, Tansy, Wintergreen, Warmseed, and Wormwood.

Oils that may Impede Concentration

Certain situations require a high level of concentration and some essential oils are too relaxing to use in such circumstances. The following oils may make it hard for you to concentrate and you should avoid them as a diffuser or having aromatherapy with these oils before such a situation:

Benzoin, Carnation, Chamomile, Geranium, Hops, Hyacinth, Lavender, Mace, Marjoram, Linden Blossom, Neroli, Nutmeg, Ormenis Flower, Petitgrain, Valerian, Spilenard, Vetiver, Ylang-Ylang, and Sandalwood.

Oils which you Must Avoid If you Have Cancer

Many cancer patients believe in alternate therapy such as aromatherapy, which they claim, give them a sense of relaxation and help them to feel good, reduce stress or depression, and soothe their senses. While many experts believe in the benefits of using essential oils with cancer patients there always recommend using them with care and after consulting a medical practitioner. To ensure safety with using essential oils with chemotherapy, experts strongly recommend following the general guidelines:

- Use essential oils in massage up to two days before chemotherapy treatment.
- Avoid using essential oils for nine to ten days after chemotherapy
- Use a low dose of essential oils during chemotherapy, reducing it to two drops per ounce of carrier oil or lotion
- If the client does not have cardiac problems or is not using chemotherapy drug 5FU, peppermint can be inhaled
- Ginger can reduce clotting time although it is a good essential oil for relieving nausea

During radiation therapy essential oils with phototoxic content should be avoided. Radiation therapy causes skin problems and extreme burning, anything which you are applying tot e skin should be clinically approved by a medical expert and carefully evaluated. Patients with skin cancer are also advised to avoid phototoxic oils as they may cause darkening of skin or make it ultra-sensitive to certain lights. It also worsens skin sensitivity and the most common phototoxic oils to avoid are:

Lemon, Bergamot, Angelica, Lime, Grapefruit, Orange, Mandarin, Tagete, Verbena

Other oils which can irritate or sensitize skin and should be avoided by person undergoing radiation therapy or those who have skin cancer are:

Cinnamon bark, Fig Leaf, Verbena, Caraway, Dill Seed, Peppermint, Ylang Ylang

Skin Irritation

For those individuals who have sensitive skin, certain essential oils should be used with care and precaution, as they are more likely to cause skin irritation or sensitization than other normal oils. Oils which can cause an irritation to your skin are:

Basil, Benzoin, Birch, Black Pepper, Cassia, Clove, Cinnamon, Lemongrass, Lemon, Oregano, Peppermint, Pine, Pimento Berry, Lemon Verbena, Tagetes, Red Thyme, and Wintergreen.

Certain essential oils can cause a rash, blotching or itching to the skin even when diluted. The following oils should also be avoided in this regard:

Costus, Elecampane, Cinnamon Bark, Fennel, Cassia

Using Oils to Treat Hypertension/Blood Pressure

Hypertension a condition that refers to high blood pressure is a cause of heart disease but it is preventable. Certain essential oils because of their properties such as hypertensive (an agent that lowers blood pressure), sedative, and calming can help in treating hypertension. The most commonly used essential oils for this purpose are **Ylang Ylang, Sweet Marjoram, and Lavender.** These oils are a great remedy for high blood pressure that you make changes to your lifestyle and diet.

Other oils, which are effective in treating stress or tension, which is usually associated with the condition of high blood pressure, are **Roman Chamomile, Neroli, Frankincense, and Bergamot.**

The benefits of these essential oils can be incorporated into daily life by inhalation, massage, or topical application. However, before using these oils make sure to check with your medical practitioner

Deciding on Dilution Levels and Different ways of Using Essential Oils

The natural form of many essentials oils is dense and highly concentrated. Its undiluted application to skin may harm certain skin types. It should be properly diluted to make it mild enough for safe application.

Dilution levels may differ depending upon its usage, purpose, individual health, age and other health-related conditions. Similarly, the way it is being used also affects its quantity and dilution.

Here is a guide to different uses of ways of using essential oils:

Add essential oils to your bath

Direct application of undiluted oil can irritate or damage the skin and mucus membranes. To avoid any risks, the safest way is to add it to your bath. It is a wonderful way to relax and steal an escape from the stressful and hectic lifestyle. While you are bathing, its winding aroma and sweet smell will sooth your senses and frayed nerves. For an added effect, light up a candle and turn off all other lights.

Depending on your skin type, you can add up to 20 drops of an essential oil. It will do wonders for people who want an effective solution against cellulite. This natural way of reducing weight is much better alternative of lasers, surgeries, synthetic creams and other electrical procedures. You will not only look attractive, but will also feel beautiful. Essential oils mixed in your bath, will eventually reduce fatty cells from your body. It is an easy-to-use every day treatment that will give you long term benefits.

Mixing 5 drops of juniper berry with 5 drops of orange and 5 drops of cypress will form an effective anti-cellulite oil blend. It will significantly reduce water retention in your body, thus making you slimmer and smarter! You can also consider mixing the oil in a small amount of bath bubbles before pouring it into the bathtub. Be careful, for some oils can quickly evaporate, therefore it is best that you add the oil in the last few minutes of the bath.

Caution:

Do not use more than 4 drops of oil for elder people and children between the ages of 4 and 12. Whereas, pregnant women and children between the ages of 1 to 4 should use only 2 drops of oil (per bath).

Cellulite Baths

Fill in the bathtub with lukewarm water. Pour in 150ml of apple cider vinegar. Pour in measured essentials oils and disperse it in the water using your hand. Enter the bath and soak for about half an hour. For soothing the skin, add in a tablespoon of olive oil. Do not worry if the water starts to feel a little warmer as some oils naturally have a warming effect.

Oils that effectively fight cellulite includes Lemon, Ginger, Orange, Sandalwood, Citronella, Grapefruit and Rosemary.

Using Burner or Vaporizer

Essential oils can also be used by means vaporizers, burners, diffusers and light-bulb rings. These highly concentrated plant oils have a strong aroma and fragrance that can be spread throughout a space when heated. It directly affects your appetite through body's sensory organs.

Although, on an average, 6 drops of oil should be enough, but the amount of oil to be added may be different depending on various factors:

- The type of diffuser, vaporizer, or burner used
- Age of people who are present in or around the room
- Size of the room
- Type of oil

When using a tea-light burner and metal light-bulb ring, oil should always be mixed with a few drops of water in order to prevent it from burning. However, in case of porcelain light-bulb rings, it is not necessary to dilute the oil. Make sure you don't drop oil directly onto the light-bulb. Some humidifiers available in the market have an opening through which oils can be poured in – but here, adding water in the reservoir can prove to be a hazard.

Before using any essential oil in a nebulizer, kindly review the product instructions on the package or consult a doctor if you are suffering from any medical condition.

Caution:

Should you use diffusers with candles, be careful, as some essential oils are flammable.

Essential oils in Lotions; Anti Fattening Creams

One of the many uses of essential oils can be in form of homemade lotions and creams. Making it is very simple; all you have to do is dilute or mix it in an un-perfumed cream or lotion.

Many people find the oiliness of these oils rather annoying and irritating. To make it feel non-oily on the skin, experts have come up with a creative solution. When these oils are mixed with a plain base cream, the strong therapeutic characteristics transfer to the cream, making it an anti-fattening cream. It is an excellent solution. It is an excellent solution for people who naturally have an oily skin.

One problem with oil is the fact that it does not only make the application part sticky, but also leaves stains on clothes and everything else that comes in contact with the skin. You can apply it to various body parts and comfortably go to work also. Un-perfumed creams can be easily purchased from your local pharmacy or departmental store.

Refer to the following chart for guidelines regarding the cream or lotion preparation:

Age/Medical Condition	Base Lotion or Cream	Essential Oil
Pregnant	50g	4 drops
Children under 1 year	50g	2 drops
Children between 1 to 4 years	50g	4 drops
Children between 4 to 12 years	50g	10 drops
Adults (12 to 65)	50g	20 drops
Elderly People (65 years+)	50g	10drops

For optimum results, make sure that the oil and cream are vigorously mixed. Also, please check if you are allergic to any substance found in the cream or the oil. Store the mixture in a cool dry place.

Adding essential oil to a massage blend

Aromatherapy became popular as scientists began to unleash the hidden healing properties of essential oils. It is now an independent branch of alternative medicine, which is being used by doctors throughout the globe. While it is known for its soothing and healing effects on body, mind, and spirit, it is also effective at weight loss.

Now that there is enough clinical evidence to support these claims, many massage practitioners have started using these oils as a part of their therapy. While it's direct application affects body's metabolism rate, its physiological effects help in calming the tensed nerves through inhalation.

It is a new ray of hope for people who had almost given up on their fatty bulges. Weight loss is often correlated with the term 'perspiration' and 'hard-work,' however, your views are about to change because now you can lose weight as you relax. Where massage itself is considered a retreat, the addition of essential oils takes the satisfaction to a whole other level.

Oil Blend for Effective Weight Loss

Follow these steps to make your own natural massage oil blend. Many men and women have benefited from this special weight loss recipe and you might be the next one!

In a measuring cup, add 2 ounces of any carrier oil. Some known carrier oils include walnut, jojoba, hazelnut, sweet almond, avocado, and coconut oil. While you can choose any of these, but experts recommend using sweet almond oil for it is rich in many minerals like magnesium and calcium as well as vitamins like D and E. Now add and combine5 drops each of lemon, cypress, and grapefruit essential oils. Transfer the mixture in a clean and dried glass bottle, tightly put the lid on, and shake well until all ingredients are blended. Using a few drops of oil, massage your abdomen or any other desired area in circular motion. For best results, apply daily or twice a day.

20 Proven Essential Oils: Say Hello to a Beautiful You

Grapefruit Essential Oil

This wonderfully fragrant oil is extracted from a glossy leaved tree called Citrus Paradisi. Although its origin is from, but now it is widely being cultivated through United States and Brazil. The color of this oil may vary between pale yellow and light ruby depending on the region where it is planted.

Helping with Weight Loss and Other Medical Conditions

Having a high content of vitamin C, it is known for its fat-dissolving properties. It prevents bloating by stopped water retention in the body, thus stopping any extra fat accumulation.

Its usefulness is beyond just fighting cellulite, it promotes positive thoughts, encourages emotions, evokes senses, revives tired muscles, and boosts digestion system. It gives a strong protection against cold and flu in winters. It also used in various herbal cosmetics as it effectively removes oil from skin pores, leaving it thoroughly cleansed and acne-free. Many skin specialists now recommend it to people who have an extremely oily skin.

Healing properties

Therapists widely use it for its natural healing properties like antibacterial, anti-infectious, antidepressant, diuretic, and lymphatic stimulant. This is one reason why it is widely used for medicinal purposes.

Home Fragrance Oils

The vapors of this oil can be used to treat addiction, headache, hangover, depression, and mental fatigue. No wonder why it is one of the hottest selling products of companies who offer scented burners and vaporizers.

Massage or Bath Oil

It effectively fights cellulite when used as massage oil. For best results, pour a few drops in bath water, as it will easily blend in. While it is battling with your fat deposits, it's refreshing scent will fuel your energy lost by cold, flu, and physical exertion.

Application as a Moisturizer

The vitamin C found in grapefruit essential oil works both ways: it dries out excess oil and fat, while nourishing the skin to regain its natural balance of moisture and elasticity.

Creating a Blend of Essential Oils

Many people like to blend and mix two fragrances together to create a new scent or achieve better results. Try mixing it with lavender, basil and bergamot for an exceptionally wonderful effect on your senses.

Precautions

Even though grapefruit oil is completely toxic free, it may cause irritation if skin is exposed to direct sun light right after the treatment. When you buy a bottle of this essential oil, mark the opening date as it should not be used after 6 months of opening date.

Allspice Essential Oil

Allspice (also known as Jamaica Pepper) oil is extracted from a plant called Pimenta Dioica. As the name suggests, this tree is native to West Indies and South America where farmers take care of it for three years before it starts bearing fruit. Mainly obtained by the leaf of the plant, this yellow colored oil has a clove like strong smell.

Helping with Weight Loss and Other Medical Conditions

You might not have heard of this oil in aromatherapy, but due to its therapeutic properties, this warming oil effectively combats fat deposits and reduces the risk of cardiovascular diseases that are caused by obesity. It also treats cramps, indigestion, flatulence and nausea.

Healing Properties

Due to the natural curative properties this essential oil, it is wise idea to always keep it at home. It serves the purpose of antioxidant, muscle relaxant, painkiller, antiseptic, stimulant and tonic.

Home Fragrance Oils

When you have allspice essential oil, a few drops in the oil burner will remove all Monday blues. Whether it is a bout of mood swings or a bad day at work, its fresh, warm, and spicy aroma will ease the stress in no time.

Massage or Bath Oil

A massage (using few drops) of allspice oil on chest can considerably cure and ease the harsh effects of infection, cold and muscle spasm. It is excellent for people who are suffering from arthritis, rheumatism, congestion, stiffness, and cough.

Creating a Blend of Essential Oils

Although you may blend it with any other available essential oil, it blends perfectly, however, with ginger, orange, lavender and geranium.

Precautions

Allspice is usually diluted more than other essential oils as its strong natural chemical composition might irritate the mucus membrane causing skin irritation.

Basil Essential Oil

This oil comes from a herb that is native to Pacific Island and Tropical Asia, called, 'OcimumBasilicum.' Due to its various uses and benefits, it is now widely grown throughout Europe and United States. The plant is also known as sweet basil. This greenish-yellow colored oil has a watery viscosity that offers a light aroma.

Helping with Weight Loss and Other Medical Conditions

This is one the most popular aromatherapy essential oils, especially to help reduce weight. Its crisp smell stimulates mind that generally clarity of thoughts and increased focus. When working out, it clean aroma will help you concentrate more. It also eases fever and sinus congestion. If you regularly suffer from asthma and sinus infections, you should consider carry a bottle in your car or handbag. Research and other experimental studies have revealed its positive implications on the treatment of respiratory tract.

By helping the body release unwanted fat toxins, basil oils can help in reducing weight. Stress, which is another cause of obesity, can also be treated as its rich aroma alleviates signs of fatigue and mental strain.

Due to the natural Emmenagogue properties of herb, it is a proven home remedy to cure and normalize menstrual abnormalities such as disturbed cycles and scanty periods. Such hormonal disturbances are one of the major reasons of obesity and overweight.

Its various other uses include:

- Calming down the condition of nausea and vomiting
- Reduce the amount of uric acid in blood
- Controlling acne
- Treatment of insect bites

Religious Practices

Being a herb that is sacred to Hindu Gods, it is highly valued in India. It's a ritual to chew its leaves before participating in any religious affair. It is believed to possess protective qualities due to which it is often applied by Hindu believers. It is also a major ingredient in many Chinese and Ayurvedic medicines.

Healing Properties

Its medicinal properties include antidepressant, anti-venomous, diaphoretic, carminative, febrifuge, antispasmodic, digestive, emmenagogue, cephalic, expectorant, insecticide, stomachic, nervine, sudorific, tonic, analgesic and stimulant.

Home Fragrance Oils

In vapor therapy, basil oil can be used for migraines, headaches and to help increase concentration and clear the mind.

Massage or Bath Oil

5to 6drops of basil oil in warm water works miracles when it comes to relieving pain caused by gout, arthritis, muscular strain and menstrual pains.

Creating a Blend of Essential Oils

This essential oil compliments many other natural oils such as Bergamot, Ginger, Black Pepper, Grapefruit, Fennel, Lavender, Neroli and Lemon.

Precautions

Although this oil is highly beneficial, it should never be used by pregnant women and children under 16 years. If used in excess amounts, it may have staggering effects. Also, be careful if you a sensitive skin as it can cause dermis irritation.

Bergamot Essential Oil

This citrus-scented essential oil is extracted from a tree that bears a fruit known as Chinese Bitter Orange. The tree is known as Citrus Aurantium Var. Bergamot essential oil has a watery viscosity and the natural color may vary between yellow and green.

Helping with Weight Loss and Other Medical Conditions

The fresh smell of this plant oil oozes positive energy and happy feelings. This effectively cures depression, which is one of the vital causes of obesity. It is excellent for people who tend to eat more when they are emotionally disturbed.

It is one of most widely used aromatherapy oils as it is not just an anti-cellulite agent; it also treats diseases like urinary tract infections, digestion problems, and spleen issues. Doctors have also begun suggesting it for treatment of acne, oily skin, acne, cold sores, and eczema.

A Treasure for People who are Overweight

The emotional setback of not looking good often results in lack of confidence, shyness, and consistent depression. Since they are most of the time irritated, they often find it difficult to exercise, which is an essential part of a healthy weight loss program. Bergamot oil is a priceless gift for such individuals because it returns their lost confidence and boosts their morale.

Healing Properties

Bergamot oil has many natural therapeutic properties like antidepressant, calmative, antiseptic, deodorant, antibiotic, digestive, anti-spasmodic and febrifuge.

Home Fragrance Oils

When it comes to losing weight, the most important thing that you need is 'willpower.' However, unfortunately, overweight people are already prone to stress and this time consuming procedure can be very frustrating. Therefore, they need some kind of energy to keep on going with their mission. Thanks to bergamot essential oil vapor therapy, you can get rid of depression and a pessimist attitude. It also helps in treating cold, flu and other respiratory problems.

Massage or Bath Oil

Massage of a few drops of this essential oil can treat compulsive eating disorder. It can also be blended with other oils and used in a bath for maximum benefits against skin problems, colds and flu, stress, postnatal depression, anxiety and depression. It particularly helps in treating anorexia nervosa, which is a kind of eating order that causes rapid weight gain.

Application as a Moisturizer

It is a wonderful ingredient to be used with an un-fragrant lotion. Due to its anti-bacterial properties, it is excellent for healing wounds, cuts, acne, chicken pox and scabies.

Creating a Blend of Essential Oils

While all essentials oils can be blended with one another, but a specific mixture of oils give enhanced results. Try mixing it with jasmine, orange, sandal wood and black pepper for a special aroma. It also goes well with cypress, rosemary, clary sage, nutmeg and mandarin.

Precautions

Be careful when using on sensitive skin as it may cause a burning sensation. Avoid exposing your skin to sunlight after its application for its high content of bergaptene may result in photo-toxicity. It is advisable to keep out of the sun if this oil is used on the skin.

Black Pepper Essential Oil

It is extracted out of a plant known as Piper nigrum, which belongs to the Piperaceae family. It is native to the subcontinent and Southeast Asia, however, due to its benefits; oil is now being made in US and UK also.

Helping with Weight Loss and Other Medical Conditions

The spicy and warn sensation of this oil significantly increases blood circulation which in turn helps in reducing weight. Its warmth also reduces joint pains and sore muscles, which is a common health issue caused by excess body weight. Its wild aroma helps in normalizing the digestion system and kidney function.

Black pepper oil is an effective treatment for nervous tension, colds, flu, muscular aches, and knee joint pain. All of these health conditions are discouraging factors for a person who is trying to reduce weight.

Healing Properties

The curative properties of this historic oil consist of antitoxic, digestive, analgesic, febrifuge, antiseptic, diaphoretic, antispasmodic and aphrodisiac.

Home Fragrance Oils

Black pepper oil vapor therapy can help create ambiance that screams 'don't give up.'

Massage or Bath Oil

It can be used as massage oils or bath oil to help increase the blood circulation. An improved circulation itself heals many health conditions including pains and sores.

Creating a Blend of Essential Oils

This plant oil particularly goes well with bergamot, lemon, ginger, lavender, sandalwood, fennel, coriander, grapefruit and clove.

Precautions

Excess use of black pepper essential oil should be avoided by pregnant women as it may over-stimulate the kidneys.

Clove Bud Essential Oil

Clove oil can be extracted from the Eugenia caryophyllataplant's stem, buds and leaves. It was traditionally used by the Chinese, Romans and Greeks as a mouthwash before speaking to Emperors and high command officials. It was used as a shield against contagious diseases like plaque.

Helping with Weight Loss and Other Medical Conditions

Although clove oil is not a famous aromatherapy ingredient, but is highly effective for seasonal ailments and obesity related diseases. This beneficial herb oil is readily available at all pharmacy and departmental stores. Keep it in your medicine wardrobe at all times, as it is a naturally healing substance. It can be used to stop infections and bacteria that cause acne. I also helps with cuts, burns, bruises, mouth sores, toothache and arthritis.

Remember that clove oil is valuable for how it aids and boosts your body and mind to continue the struggle towards weight loss. Use it as a support system and not as a complete therapy for losing excess bad weight

Healing Properties

Clove oil is known for its therapeutic properties such as carminative, disinfectant, analgesic, anti-infectious, antiseptic, stimulant, and antispasmodic.

Home Fragrance Oils

When used in an oil burner, clove oil can help you get rid of depression and dizziness that might be stopping you from a daily workout routine. It also strengthens memory through improved blood circulation.

Pour a few drops of oils onto a cotton ball and place it in your wardrobe. I will not only make the closet fragrant, but will also keep fish moths away.

Massage or Bath Oil

Clove oil massage can stimulate metabolism rate, which helps in reducing excess body fat.

Application as a Moisturizer

For people who have an extremely oily skin, it is best to dilute the oil in a cream or lotion. While its effectiveness on cellulite will remain the same, its form will be much milder.

Creating a Blend of Essential Oils

Due to its strong aroma, its best to blend it with oils that have a sweeter scent such as cinnamon, ginger, basil, lavender and clary sage.

Precautions

Clove oil should always be handled with care, as it is highly potent. When being used with creams, lotions, or shampoos, the dilution level must be less than 1%. Pregnant women should avoid using this oil as it increases skin sensitivity and may cause irritation.

Mouthwash

Add a drop or two into your mouthwash bottle for additional protection against germs and a longer lasting fresh breath.

Coriander Seed Essential Oil

This spicy and warm-scented oil is extracted from a plant known as Coriandrumsativum. This colorless substance is one of the most widely most aromatherapy product all over the world.

Helping with Weight Loss and Other Medical Conditions

Apply a few drops of diluted oil can significantly reduce mood swings, anxiety, digestive disorders, flu, cold and nervous weakness. Once all of these physiological and psychological symptoms are gone, you will automatically feel good about yourself. These positive inner emotions help in reducing weight. Its warming effect on the body will uplift the mind and improve circulation glandular system. It also detoxifies the body to eliminate toxins and fluid wastes that cause obesity.

Healing Properties

Coriander is enriched with many therapeutic properties such as digestive, antispasmodic, analgesic, carminative, depurative, fungicidal, deodorant, carminative, stimulant and lipolytic.

Home Fragrance Oils

Inhaling its vapors can help in treating eating disorders.

Massage or bath oil

Another way to use it is to dilute it in a small shampoo bottle and mix it in the bath, or by simply applying it to your body in form of massage. Do not forget to dilute it in a carrier oil. It will help in detoxifying the body, thus flushing out bad fat cells.

Application as Moisturizer

It can be added to a lotion or a mild face cream to directly treat the affected area and problem. You will not only get a healthier and clearer looking skin, but also stay away from problems such as anxiety, migraine, joint pains, muscular spasms and digestive problems.

Creating a Blend of Essential Oils

This anti-cellulite essential oil can be blended with lemon, orange, ginger, grapefruit, bergamot and cinnamon for exceptional changes in emotional stability and clearer thoughts.

Precautions

Coriander is one of the very few oils that is not associated with any contra-indications or side effects.

Cumin Seed Essential Oil

This Mediterranean herb oil is extracted from Cuminumcyminum, which is a small herb that grows about 50cm high. Its history dates back to the biblical times when it was mainly used it for headaches digestion problems. While this tasteful herb is generally only associated with Indian and Middle Eastern cuisines, it is also a widely used ingredient in Spanish and Mexican kitchens.

Helping with Weight Loss and Other Medical Conditions

It is an amazing weight loss product for all those who wish to have the perfect body shape. It stimulates bad fat deposits in the body in four effective ways. It breaks down stored fat, reduces water retention and bloating, increases metabolism and controls cravings for carbs.

Recently, a study revealed that that antioxidants found in cumin in are far more effective than the ones found in Vitamin C. Health professionals believe that its strong antioxidant content may aid in fighting cancer.

After using this, you will notice significant changes in your metabolism, energy, complexion and hair loss. Expert aroma therapists strongly recommend using this miracle herb as it will not only make you skinnier, but is also good for general health.

Healing Properties

Chefs throughout the world love cumin for its strong flavor, but its impressive health properties have attracted many therapists also. Some of its most prominent healing properties include Emmenagogue, antitoxic, digestive, bactericidal, anti-spasmodic, nervine, antiseptic, carminative, stimulant and tonic.

Home Fragrance Oils

The vapors of cumin oil can reduce the craving experienced by people who either have lack of energy, or are just habitual of nibbling. It also helps in treating digestive problems.

Massage or Bath oil

It may be added to the bath if you desire maximum results in a minimum time.

Creating a Blend of Essential Oils

This warming oil blends perfectly with lavender, allspice, grapefruit and angelica.

Precautions

Due to its overwhelming scent, it should be used carefully for people who are allergic to strong smell might get a headache. It is best to start the therapy with a small amount of oil, and gradually increase its usage, as body gets immune of its smell. Although it is non-sensitizing, non-irritant, and non-toxic, but it does not suggest that it is safe to put it on before taking a sunbath.

Pregnant women and people with sensitive skin should not use it.

Dill Essential Oil

This calming botanical oil is extracted from Anethumsowa through the process of drying and compressing. Its history can be traced back to the medieval ages when it was thought to have magical healing remedial powers. After centuries, when researchers conducted studies, it was revealed that magic was merely the scientific curative properties that were extremely effective at healing.

Helping with Weight Loss and Other Medical Conditions

One of the biggest causes of weight gain is imbalances and disturbances emotional and mental wellbeing. There may be a combination of other related components also, however, these two are the basic factors that promote obesity. This is perhaps the reason why many people either re-gain weight or go off the track in maintaining a fat-free diet. Dill oil plays its part here – it revives senses, giving a clearer mind with more positive and constructive thoughts.

Other uses of dill oil in aromatherapy are aimed at combating digestion problems including constipation and flatulence.

Brigham Young University conducted a study in 2003 that revealed an incredible fact about dill essential oil. Research suggests that it provides 56.6% inhibition against prostate cancer.

Healing Properties

Dill essential oil has therapeutic properties such as disinfectant, carminative, sudorific, antispasmodic, sedative, galactagogue, digestive and stomachic.

Home Fragrance Oils

Dill vapor therapy is known to revive the senses and nervous tension as well as indigestion.

Massage or Bath oil

Massage your feet with a few drops of dill essential oil to experience health benefits like improved blood circulation, healthy digestion system, increased metabolism and enhanced memory.

Creating a Blend of Essential Oils

While this oil may be blended with any other essential oil, it smells and works best with nutmeg, bergamot and citrus oils like lemon and orange.

Precautions

Although there are no proven side effects of dill essential oil as it is non-sensitizing, non-toxic and non-irritant, but it must not be used by pregnant woman. Once the baby is delivered and mother has recovered from the post-delivery complications, it is safe to be used during nursing.

Fennel Essential Oil

Fennel essential oil refers to the plant oil extracted from Foeniculumvulgare var. dulce. It is a biennial herb that has feathery leaves and grows up to 2 meters high. Although it is a Mediterranean plant but it is widely being cultivated across the globe. It is important to note that Fennel basically has two species, one is sweet and the other one is bitter. In aromatherapy, the sweet fennel essential oil is used as it is very gentle.

Helping with Weight Loss and Other Medical Conditions

In ancient times, it was used by Chinese, Indians, Romans, Greeks and Egyptians for various health remedies. Greek health experts were the first to unleash its diuretic properties that can help a person lose excess weight and maintain a healthy digestion system. Since this herb is an amazing weight loss product, Greeks called it "Marathron" which means 'to grow thin.'

Looking at the Egyptian pyramids, don't we wonder how did people manage to move such huge rocks without any machinery? It might be hard to believe but Egyptian workers were in habit of using fennel to suppress their appetite while maintaining the same levels of energy during hardships.

It also cures a huge array of other health problems such as cholesterol, obesity, cardiac diseases, digestive problems, acne and extremely oily skin conditions and wrinkles caused by lack of collagen. Romans believed that using fennel would result in longevity, improved strength and enhanced courage, because of this it was frequently given to soldiers and athletes. In India, it is still being used as a home remedy to ease colic in newborns.

Healing Properties

This magical herb is known to have healing properties like laxative, diuretic,aperitif,stomachic,emmenagogue,antiseptic,carminative,vermifuge, stimulant, antispasmodic, galactagogue, expectorant, depurative and tonic.

Home Fragrance Oils

Vapor therapy of dill essential oil is highly effective at obesity. It stimulates the body for better blood circulation causing fatty deposits to burn off. Here is a secret for why you will surely try it – it tones out the skin to make you look at least 10 years younger than your actual age.

Massage or bath oil

To slim down your bloated stomach, create a massage blend or used its diluted form in bath. While it beautifies you externally, it will also fix any internal abnormalities including digestive problems, excess water retention, constipation, and enhanced energy,

Application as Moisturizer

When mixed in a base cream, fennel oil can be applied to face to resolving skin related issues including dull complexion, acne caused by oily skin, and wrinkles caused by decreased skin elasticity.

Creating a Blend of Essential Oils

It blends wonderfully with lavender, sandalwood, geranium and rose.

Precautions

Sweet fennel carries highly potent content due to which it should not be used frequently in large doses. Its repetitive usage may result in a narcotic or addiction effect. It contains a large percentage of trans-anethole, which may be harmful for pregnant women, nursing mothers and patients with estrogen linked cancers. Remember that all of these benefits are related to sweet fennel essential oil. Bitter fennel must not be applied to skin under any circumstances.

Ginger Essential Oil

This Ginger essential oil is extracted from a perennial herb called Zingiberaceaeofficinale. The plant grows approximately 3 to 4 feet high. Its use in the field of medicine can be traced back to ancient times and its evidence if sound in both Chinese and Sanskrit historical texts. The name of the herb itself refers to a district in India, Gingi, where a special kind of tea is produced which treats stomach upsets.

Helping with Weight Loss and Other Medical Conditions

Ginger oil can give your metabolism a big boost. Although it does not directly burn the fat, but its stimulation effect can help with weight loss. It's naturally found chemicals cut down fat deposits that are stored in your body in form of cellulite.

This can help you lose weight and cut the fat deposits in your body through lipolysis. It encourages cells to discharge the toxic fat remains. In addition to that, its strong refreshing aroma also helps in keeping you motivated to overcome any emotional hindrances that might stop you from following a diet plan or continue exercising.

Healing Properties

Ginger is beneficial in many ways as it holds an array of therapeutic properties such as laxative,stimulant,antispasmodic,rubefacient,carminative,expectorant,anti-emetic,stomachic,antiseptic,bactericidal and tonic.

Home Fragrance Oils

Vapor therapy of ginger can help with emotional and physiological symptoms like lethargy, catarrh, flu, cold, loss of libido or sexual desire and feeling of loneliness.

Massage or bath oil

For patients who are suffering from arthritis and joint pain, using ginger essential oil in the bath can be a source of ease and comfort. Similarly, a massage of blended oils can improve poor blood circulation.

Creating a Blend of Essential Oils

Since ginger essential oil has an overpowering scent, no other oil's smell will change its aroma much. For more effective results, combine it with spicy or citrus oils like sandalwood, bergamot, neroli, frankincense and rose.

Precautions

Highly concentrated oil blends may result in skin irritation. Also, be careful if you have a sensitive skin as it may cause photosensitivity.

Jasmine Essential Oil

Jasmine essential oil is extracted from an evergreen shrub called JasminumGradiflora. The name is inspired by a Persian word Yasmin. While it is indigenous to Northern India and China, but now it is being cultivated throughout the globe in suitable environments. It has floral, sweet, and exotic perfume-like scents due to which it is relatively more expensive than other essential oils. What is special about this plant is the fact that its flowers are carefully picked by experienced pickers at night only.

While Indians, Arabians and Chinese sometimes used it medicinally, at other times, they also used its star-shaped flower for ceremonial purposes. Turks used its wood while Chinese used its leaves as tea. In short, this small shrub served many purposes in different cultures and societies.

Helping with Weight Loss and Other Medical Conditions

All of us know that weight loss is never a piece of cake! It takes time, will power, and a handful of determination to stay focus with your objective. Often this frustrates people, forcing them to give up too quickly. Although jasmine oil is famous for its therapeutic properties, in reality, it does much more than that – it can turn your world into a paradise. It may sound absurd, but its sensational aroma does have a magical effect on our senses.

It deeply relaxes the senses, boosts confidence, lifts off feelings of depression, eases labor or childbirth, improves desire for intimacy, arouses sexual hormones, improves skin elasticity, sooths coughing, and reduces stretch marks caused by obesity.

Healing Properties

The health benefits of Jasmine Essential Oil can be recognized by its curative properties such as anti-depressant, parturient, antiseptic, expectorant, aphrodisiac, cicatrisant, anti-spasmodic, galactagogue and sedative.

Home Fragrance Oils

Inhaling jasmine essential oil molecules can help stabilize mood and fix disorders like emotional eating. It transmits messages to limbic system, which is a function of brain that controls emotions and the nervous system. It helps in treating menstrual cramps, stress, depression, and anxiety.

Massage or bath oil

Using it as bath or massage oil, both are effective because when this oil is absorbed through the skin, it influences biological state, including blood pressure, immune system, heart rate, breathing, and stress levels. It is natural remedy for menopausal symptoms such as muscular and joint pain.

Application as Moisturizer

Jasmine oil helps treat dry skin and acts as a natural moisturizer to the skin, like other essential natural oils. You can apply it as a moisturizer confidently and be sure that it will not clog any pores.

To apply jasmine oil you first need to choose a carrier oil such as olive oil, borage oil, almond oil, or hemp oil. Then combine 20 drops of therapeutic jasmine oil with ½ an ounce of the carrier oil. Apply 4 to 6 drops to your skin evenly in the morning and evening, after cleansing. You can store the moisturizer in the refrigerator to keep it fresh.

Creating a Blend of Essential Oils

This floral scented oil works well with almost all other essential oils, however, the aroma produced by its combination with rose, citrus oil, sandalwood or bergamot is truly exciting.

Precautions

Although this oil is completely safe to use as it no elements that are toxic, irritant or sensitizing, but it is best to carry out a skin patch test before starting the treatment. Sometimes people have a natural energy towards a certain chemical compound, but they remain unaware, as they never encounter that substance. It should not be used by pregnant woman for it does carry a minimal amount of Emmenagogue.

Lemon Essential Oil

Extracted from the peel of Citrus limonum, lemon essential oil is widely used in aromatherapy. Along with a large number of health benefits, it provides an ultimate solution for weight loss. Did you know that in ancient Rome, lemon was a symbol denoted for Juventas, the Goddess of Youth? Continue reading to find exactly why!

Helping with Weight Loss and Other Medical Conditions

Aromatically, this natural oil has a refreshing and soothing effect on body, mind and soul. Therefore, it proves to be beneficial and useful in times of great stress, relationship crisis, work related pressures and sexual problems. It triggers positivity that stimulates senses to overcome any obstacle.

The botanical oil treatment is a promising experience for people who wish to fit in to their favorite dress without having to feel much pain. In a biological study conducted on lab rats, it was revealed that breathing in the vapors of lemon essential oil significantly reduced the fatty molecules in the body.

Healing Properties

Health benefits of lemon essential oil can be associated with its natural curative properties such as anti-anemic, vermifuge, antimicrobial, rubefacient, anti-rheumatic, hypotensive, anti-sclerotic, febrifuge, antiseptic, diaphoretic, bactericidal, diuretic, carminative, haemostatic, cicatrisantand depurative.

Home Fragrance Oils

Lemon vapor therapy has positive implications on the overall wellbeing of an individual. It addresses the main causes why a person overeats including lack of energy, stress, emotional trauma, depression and fatigue. Furthermore, breathing in lemon oil vapors increases concentration, focus and determination.

Massage or bath oil

Lemon oil can be diluted in the bath or blended with other essential oils to reduce cellulite.

Application as Moisturizer

Lemon oil mixed in a base cream can effectively treat acne and other oily skin problems. Did you know that most of the pricy oily skin care products have astringent, which is naturally found in this oil? Moreover, its antiseptic properties further reduce the damage on the skin caused by environmental pollution.

Creating a Blend of Essential Oils

Although it can be used separately also, but for a more targeted action, it is recommended that you blend it with other anti-cellulite oils. Lemon essential oil particularly blends well with oils that have a sweet or pleasant aroma including sandalwood, fennel, rose, juniper, lavender, eucalyptusand neroli.

Precautions

Although this natural substance is free of toxic elements, but some people might be allergic to its chemical composition. Conduct a skin patch test to be on a safer side. Like all citric oils, it is phototoxic even in low dilution levels. Keep the treated skin covered while going out during the day.

Lemongrass Essential Oil

This fresh smelling essential oil is extracted from Cymbopogoncitrates which is a plant native to India.

Helping with Weight Loss and Other Medical Conditions

If you want to get into the perfect body shape, this is the ultimate solution. It fights cellulite so that you can wear your favorite swimsuit without any embarrassments. Not only this, it revitalizes your body, mind and soul to clear your mind from all kind of worries and stress. It can also be used to recover from jet lag.

Healing Properties

This lemon-like scented oil has a number of healing properties including, insecticidal, analgesic, galactagogue, anti-depressant, febrifuge, antimicrobial. diuretic, antipyretic, carminative, antiseptic, deodorant, astringent, nervine, bactericidal, fungicidal and tonic.

Home Fragrance Oils

Vapor therapy of lemongrass essential oil is good for the nervous system. If you find it difficult to workout, use lemongrass essential oil to restore the energy needed for an hour of exercise.

Massage or bath oil

Lemongrass essential oil can be used as a bath oil to turn an ordinary shower into a spa treatment. It can also be massaged on to the body for additional treatment against cellulite and bad fat deposits.

Application as Moisturizer

It can play an important role in clearing cellulite. Mix it in a base cream and apply to your stomach and thighs for a more toned and firmer skin. Before sleeping, apply on the face to get of acne and other oily skin problems. Due to its antiseptic properties, it can also be applied to feet to cure infections caused by wearing shoes all day long.

Creating a Blend of Essential Oils

To create a wonderful blend of lemongrass essential oil, try mixing it with jasmine, coriander, lavender, cedarwood, tea trees, sandalwood or basil.

Precautions

Lemongrass oil can irritate a sensitive skin, so care should be taken. It should be avoided in pregnancy, due to it being a possible skin irritant.

Lime Essential Oil

Lime essential oil is obtained from Citrus aurantifolia, which is also known as sour lime. This evergreen tree is originally from Asia, but is now being cultivated in all warm countries.

Helping with Weight Loss and Other Medical Conditions

This clear smelling citrus oil has a high content of vitamin C which cellulite's worst enemy. A few drop of lime essential is good enough to cure many chronic diseases including cardiac problems, cancer and arthritis. Aroma therapists use it lift depression and treat people who are suffering from intense nervous tension.

It is frequently used in the food industry for the purpose of flavoring and adding aroma to food. Due to its soothing scent, it also used in many perfumes as one of the major ingredients.

It can be helpful for arthritis, rheumatism and poor circulation, as well as for obesity and cellulite and has an astringent and toning action to clear oily skin and acne, and also helps with herpes, insect bites and cuts.

Healing Properties

This sharp smelling liquid is known to have many medical properties such as antiseptic, restorative, antiviral, bactericidal, astringent, febrifuge, aperitif, disinfectant, tonic and haemostatic.

Home Fragrance Oils

To energize a tired mind and feel good about yourself, use lime essential oil in vapor therapy. Don't think low about yourself just because you are a few pounds heavier than others. Being overweight is not a chronic disease, it is a problem that can be resolved with some conscious efforts, exercise, good diet and a few essential oils.

Massage or bath oil

Using its diluted form as bath oil can ease joint pain, sore muscles and tensed nerves. It also helps in clearing the respiratory tract.

Application as Moisturizer

If you want to get rid of stubborn saddlebags, blend 5 drops of oil in a suitable amount of moisturizer and apply twice a day. Massage the affected area in round circular motions for about 5 minutes. The results will be astonishingly wonderful.

Creating a Blend of Essential Oils

Lime essential oil can be blended with any other oil, but for brilliant results, mix it with lavender, ylang-ylang and clary sage.

Precautions

Exposing the treated skin to sunshine may result in burning and irritation on epidermis.

Orange Essential Oil

Orange essential oil is obtained from Citrus sinensis. This evergreen tree is indigenous to China, but now it is extensively found throughout the world, usually in warm areas.

Helping with Weight Loss and Other Medical Conditions

Since obesity has become one of the major health concerns, people are usually willing to do anything to get rid of excess body weight. Orange essential oil is usually associated with the feeling of warmth and happiness. It also promotes collagen development in the skin while stimulating the lymphatic mechanism to support weight loss. Lymphatic massage can remodel the body to remove excess fluid and toxins. An unpretentious essential oil calms down tensed nerves. It has a tangy fresh smell that helps people to relax and sleep well.

Due to its strong diuretic action, it is extremely effective at balancing and controlling water retention. It does not only detoxify the body, but also strengthens the immune system and supports healthy living.

Healing Properties

This sunny-colored oil is enriched with many therapeutic properties such asantiseptic, sedative, diuretic, anti-depressant, carminative, antispasmodic, cholagogue, anti-inflammatory and tonic.

Home Fragrance Oils

Its vapor therapy is excellent for people who are obese because of sleeping disorder. It is also effective at combating cold, flu and stress, thus helping people to sleep more peacefully. Because of its sedative effect, it also helps children to sleep calmly.

Massage or bath oil

Lymphatic massage with orange essential oil improves body's ability to drain out body toxins resulting in a slimmer and thinner body shape. It works as a lymphatic stimulant that activates lymph nodes that are naturally found in every part of the body. A gentle massage strokes will help in eliminating toxins that are stored as fat in cells.

Application as Moisturizer

When used as a moisturizer, it acts a tonic for congested skin. It evens patchy and uneven skin resulting in a 'heads turning' complexion. It also helps the body to naturally form more collagen for a firmer, younger and healthier looking skin.

Creating a Blend of Essential Oils

While this natural oil can be blended with any other botanical oil, some combinations work miraculously. Try combining it with ginger, black pepper, cloves, sandalwood, cinnamon, vetiver and frankincense.

Precautions

While it is categorized as a non-sensitizing, non-toxic and non- irritant essential oil, it may have extreme phototoxic effects on some skin types. Consult a doctor or read the label of the product for details and precautions regarding its usage.

Peppermint Essential Oil

Peppermint essential oil is extracted from Menthapiperita, which is a perennial herb native to the Mediterraneanregion. It is also known as brandy mint for it has a strong menthol smell. This widely used aromatherapy oil is available at all leading pharmacies and grocery stores.

Helping with Weight Loss and Other Medical Conditions

Peppermint is an excellent aid to digestion. It has a unique way of fight cellulite and obesity – it directly affects the part of the bran that is responsible for creating the feeling of hunger. It reduces appetite and make you feel fuller when eating.

In addition to that, its cooling sensation and refreshing scent stimulates the mind which eventually results in increased focus, determination and agility. It also helps to ease muscle convulsive colon, sinus, headaches, migraine and chest congestion.

Another weight loss action of peppermint essential oil is increased metabolism and improved digestive system. Pour a few drop of essential oil on a cotton ball and inhale it for 4 to 5 minutes for increased work efficiency and vitality.

Peppermint oil can also be used to heal certain damaging emotions. Its aroma helps in reviving the mind to eliminate mental fatigue and a state of depression. It is excellent to recover from effects of shock, stress, dizziness. Lastly, it treats all kind of respiratory disorders including sinus congestion, dry coughs, pneumonia, cholera and asthma.

Healing Properties

Nature has blessed this plant with many healing properties. It can act as ananalgesic, vermifuge, anesthetic, vasoconstrictor antiseptic, sudorific, antigalactagogue, febrifuge, antiphlogistic, emmenagogue, antispasmodic, stomachic, astringent, stimulant, carminative, expectorant, cephalic, nervine, decongestant and hepatic.

Home Fragrance Oils

Vapor therapy of peppermint essential oil can be used for weight loss, improved concentration, relief from headache and better breathing.

Massage or bath oil

When used as a bath oil, it can assist with headaches, muscular pains, constipation, colic, inflamed bowel disorders, cramps, back pain, tired feet, spastic colon, mental fatigue, itchy skin, inflammations, coughs and nausea. The same affects can be achieved by means of massage.

Application as Moisturizer

Include it in a base cream to get a fresh complexion. Thanks to its vasoconstrictor properties, it reduces redness, cold down itchiness, and the appearance of blemishes caused by oily skin.

Creating a Blend of Essential Oils

To make the most of this natural oil, blend it with lemon, lavender, benzoin, rosemary and marjoram.

Precautions

It should never be used pregnant women in any form. It may prove too dangerous for the fetus. When applying on skin, keep away from eyes as it can cause burning and irritation in the pupil. It is best not to use for children under the age of 7 as its strong aroma may have adverse effects. Before using such powerful compounds, you should always conduct a skin patch test because sometimes its menthol affects causes sensitization.

Spearmint Essential Oil

Spearmint essential oil is obtained from Menthaspicata, which belongs to the family of mint plants.

Helping with Weight Loss and Other Medical Conditions

This stimulating oil is believed to boost the metabolism rate due to which it is commonly used in aromatherapy as part of weight loss program. It has a bright crisp aroma that controls sweet cravings. Once the person stops nibbling (and eating between meals), it normalizes body and thus excess weight is reduced.

Spearmint oil can also assist in nervous disorders and is dramatically effective in stimulating brain cells for increased focus and concentration. It has proven to be helpful in treating the respiratory tract, muscular aches and pains and skin problems. Since its contents are the same as peppermint, it is safe to be used by children.

A few drops of spearmint essential oil in your regular mouthwash will prevent gum infections and give you a longer lasting fresh breath.

Healing Properties

Spearmint essential oil can act as an antiseptic, stimulant, antispasmodic, insecticide, carminative, emmenagogue, cephalic and restorative.

Home Fragrance Oils

In vapor therapy, spearmint oil can be used for vomiting, colic, flatulence, headaches, migraines, nervous conditions, asthma, bronchitis, sinusitis and catarrh.

Massage or bath oil

When used as massage oil, it can help melt down the toxins stored in cells and significantly reduce cellulite.

Application as Moisturizer

For people who have an oily skin texture, this form of blend works best. Use a base cream that is less oily as additional oil will make it oilier.

Creating a Blend of Essential Oils

Spearmint essential oil blends well with Rosemary, Sandalwood, Jasmine, Basil, Bergamot and Lemon.

Precautions

Be careful when using this oil for the first time. Some people may end up with a painful headache it has a strong aroma. Remember that all minty oils should not be used by pregnant women.

Sandalwood Essential Oil

Sandalwood essential oil is obtained from Santalum album.

Helping with Weight Loss and Other Medical Conditions

Sandalwood essential oil regulates and stops stress eating. By stabilizing emotions, compulsive eating can be prevented. It will help you overcome negative thoughts and emotions that generally lead to a deep state of stress.

Healing Properties

Sandalwood essential oil is used in many herbal medicines due its therapeutic properties such as antiphlogistic, sedative, emollient, antiseptic, carminative, antispasmodic, diuretic, astringent and tonic.

Massage or bath oil

Use it a massage oil to target the fat molecules. Its sensational aroma will revive your senses, while the gentle strokes of hand will stimulate cells to improve blood circulation.

Creating a Blend of Essential Oils

Sandalwood essential oil blends perfectly well with Ylang-Ylang, Rose, Bergamot and Black Pepper.

Precautions

The oil is safe to be used by anyone, however, it is best to conduct a skin patch test before applying the product overall.

Ylang-ylang Essential Oil

Intensely sweet spicy, floral scent, Organic Ylang Ylang seduces the senses and relaxes the mind. Ylang Ylang aides in the release of possessive emotional patterns, feeling drained, and fearing wisdom.

Helping with Weight Loss and Other Medical Conditions

Its strong anti-depressant properties make it an effective tool against cellulite and excess body fat.

Healing Properties

Ylang-Ylang Essential oil is enriched with therapeutic properties such as antidepressant, sedative, antiseborrhoeic, hypotensive, antiseptic, nervine and aphrodisiac.

Precautions

It is categorized as non-irritant, non-sensitizing and non-toxic oil, yet it may result in an itchy skin as some people are naturally allergic to its chemical composition. In severe cases, it may also cause nausea and headache. It's best not to take any risk and perform a skin patch test before starting the therapy.

Essential Oil Body Wraps

Toxins can be stored in virtually any part of the body organs, blood, tissues, cells and muscles. These toxins are one the most common causes of rapid weight gain and obesity. Not only this, but also makes you sluggish, lazy and tired quickly. Even if you keep resting all day, you will still feel exhausted and worn out as if you have been working all day long. It can also make you ill and cause deep-rooted internal health problems. While drinking water is a great way to flush out these harmful deposits, you may also try an essential oil body wrap to detoxify your body. Unlike professional massage therapies, with these homemade herbal remedies, you can at least be sure about the chemicals that are used in the treatment.

In order to pull toxins out of your body, you can choose to either make a blend of various essential oils or use a combination of various naturally found substances. Remember that all essentials must be diluted in a neutral base or carrier oil before applying it.

Oils that are known to have detoxifying properties include:

- Bitter orange
- Black pepper
- Carrot seed
- Coriander
- Cypress
- Fennel
- Frankincense
- Grapefruit
- Juniper berry
- Lemon
- Nutmeg
- Parsley
- Rose

Applying and Creating a Body Wrap

Combination 1: Lemon, Juniper Berry, Fennel, Seaweed

Combination 2: Fennel, Rose, Lemon, Grapefruit

Since essential oil body wraps are often messy, it is best that you stand or lay inside the bathtub at the time of application. To prepare your skin for maximum absorption, start with taking a warm shower, as it will open up skin pores. After drying, immediately rub the oil blend all over your body. Take only a few minutes to massage your skin with oil. As soon as you finish massaging, cover or wrap yourself up with a towel. To keep yourself warm, you may use a blanket. After 45 minutes, remove the towel and end the spa treatment with a bath. You can make it a real retreat by playing a soothing music in the background.

Conclusion

These essential oils alone cannot work wonders without a support system. Aromatherapy needs to be combined with regular workouts and a healthy diet if you want permanent and maximum results.

Drink Plenty of Water

As discussed in earlier chapters, the toxic remains in our body cause fat to be accumulated. Weight loss is only possible once these harmful substances are flushed out of your body. The best way to do that is by drinking plenty of water, preferably warm. It becomes even more important especially if you already are on a diet plan. Did you know that initial weight loss is generally in the form of excess outflow of water? To prevent dehydration, you must drink at least 8 glasses of water every day. Lack of fluids in the body can hamper the fat-burning process. Exercising often results in sore muscles and joint pains. Water helps in toning the muscles and lubricating the joints for a pain-free workout.

Food and Drinks to Avoid

Stay at a distance from excessively fatty drinks and foods including meals that have a high content of protein, sugar and salt. Also, avoid drinks like tea, coffee, sugary beverages, soft drinks, highly-concentrated packed juices and energy drinks. Furthermore, next time you are going to a party, refrain from having too much alcohol as it will make you eat more than how much you need to eat.